Making the Transition to a Macrobiotic Diet

By the same author:

*An Introduction
to Macrobiotics*

Our Food, Our Future

Making the
Transition to a
Macrobiotic Diet

Carolyn Heidenry

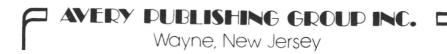
AVERY PUBLISHING GROUP INC.
Wayne, New Jersey

The publisher does not advocate the use of any particular diet program, but believes the information presented in this book should be available to the public. Because there is always some risk involved, the author and publisher are not responsible for any adverse effects or consequences resulting from the use of any of the suggestions in this book. Please do not use the book if you are unwilling to assume the risk. Feel free to consult a qualified health professional. It is a sign of wisdom, not cowardice, to seek a second or third opinion.

Cover design by Martin Hochberg and Rudy Shur
In-House Editor Jacqueline Balla
Typeset by ACS Graphic Services, Fresh Meadows, NY

Library of Congress Cataloging-in-Publication Data

Heidenry, Carolyn.
   Making the transition to a macrobiotic diet.

   Bibliography: p.
   Includes index.
   1. Macrobiotic diet.   I. Title.
RM235.H45   1987   613.2'6   86-32291
ISBN 0-89529-363-3

Printed in the United States of America

10   9   8   7   6

Contents

Acknowledgements

I am greatly indebted to Paolo Antognetti, whose guidance, assistance, and advice were so essential to the original 1984 production and publication of this book.

Special thanks also go to Patrick McDermott and Jacqueline Balla for the many excellent comments and suggestions they offered for this second and revised edition.

Preface

There was a time, not so very long ago, when people who ate health foods were regarded as mildly eccentric or, at the very least, overly protective of their health. In recent years, however, this attitude has largely changed, no doubt because of the rising incidence of degenerative diseases and other public health problems. In fact, protecting one's health through a wholesome diet has now become more of a necessity than a pleasant option. Consequently, many people are modifying their diets in some way, in order to counterbalance the effects of impure air and water, junk food, and sedentary "push-button" lifestyles.

Making this change to a better diet can be somewhat difficult at first, considering the overwhelming number of unwholesome foods on the market today. It is a step that entails a bigger adjustment than we might at first realize, for it affects something we do three times every day— each week, each month, each year. Therefore, this book is designed for those who are accustomed to a typical diet of hamburgers, soft drinks, and ice cream and who want to protect their health by improving the quality of their food.

The suggestions offered in this book have been drawn from both my own experience as well as the experiences of many friends. My initial attempt at improving my diet failed, for I tried to go immediately from donut breakfasts and TV dinners to a diet of whole grains and vegetables. Fortunately I made a second attempt, this time with success, because I learned to be patient and to take things one step at a time. In the long run, this proved to be the better route.

Few things are as important as changing your diet gradually, especially if your previous diet was particularly poor, as mine was. In fact, the worse your previous diet was, the slower your transition to a more wholesome diet should be. Those who already practice relatively sensible eating habits may find that they can make a much more rapid transition to a natural and wholesome macrobiotic diet.

Although the suggestions presented in this book may not be applicable to everyone, I think they do reflect the experiences of many people who begin a macrobiotic diet, with slight variations. It should be pointed out, however, that the following advice is not necessarily appropriate for someone who is seriously ill. Those who find themselves faced with such a challenge are obliged to muster greater resolve and to exercise greater control than the average person. Fortunately, such efforts can be very effective in alleviating and reversing disorders of all kinds, when made in a positive and supportive atmosphere. In such cases, however, guidance from qualified macrobiotic teachers or counselors is necessary. This book, on the other hand, was written for those who are *not* seriously ill, but who are simply interested in taking the necessary measures likely to prevent such an occurrence.

As simple and brief as it is, I hope this book will be useful in helping others to make the transition from a chaotic and disorderly modern diet to a more balanced, grain-based one—like the one that was traditionally used by mankind. We appear to be on the verge of a renaissance in health awareness and dietary consciousness, arising from a growing perception of the decline in public health. It is clear to many that this decline is largely a result of the inexpensive, mass-produced, artificial foods so prevalent today.

This book is Part Two of a three-part series on the subject of macrobiotics, in which I set out to answer some basic questions about this "new" (yet really very old) method of health care. The first of this series, *An Introduction to Macrobiotics*, explains, in an elementary way, what the macrobiotic diet is, and where and how it began. This volume, Part Two, contains various recommendations and suggestions on how to begin a macrobiotic diet, which many feel is the best of all natural food diets. Volume Three, *Our Food, Our Future,* deals with the question of why macrobiotics is so important to our declining society and why, more than ever before, it is becoming so necessary.

I would like to dedicate this book to all those who have, in some way, contributed to the development of macrobiotics, both past and present—whomever and wherever they may be.

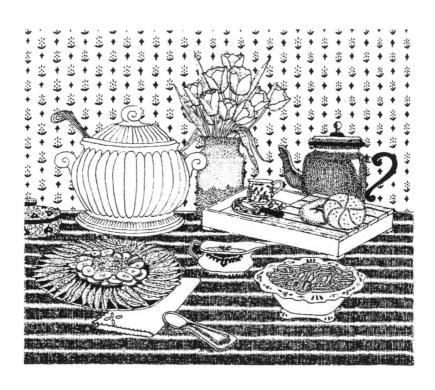

1

Choosing, Combining, & Cooking

Eating is much like any other activity, such as exercising, breathing, or singing. It can be done in such a way that it brings about beneficial and desirable results, or in a way that brings about detrimental and undesirable ones. We all know (or we may *think* we know) how to exercise and how to breathe, and we can all more or less sing. Similarly, we all know, from the moment we are born, how to *eat*.

But we do not always breathe in the best possible way, such as when we take shallow, rapid breaths instead of slow, deep ones. Likewise, we may sing with less than optimal results, due to a lack of proper training and practice. We may also exercise incorrectly or even dangerously, such as when we pull a muscle or overtax our hearts.

This also applies to the way we eat. When we eat correctly, with proper guidance, we can obtain very beneficial effects—effects which are very different from those that result from careless eating habits. By chewing our food well, and selecting and preparing our food correctly, we can reap immediate improvements in our health and well-being. This is the great value of a macrobiotic approach to diet and nutrition. It teaches the proper way to eat consistent with the climate in which you live, so that you can live the healthiest life possible.

There are three main points to consider in a macrobiotic diet, each of which will be discussed separately. These are: a. how foods are *chosen;* b. how foods are *combined;* and c. how foods are *cooked.*

CHOOSING FOODS

The macrobiotic approach to diet includes a wide variety of delicious and nutritious foods. The companion volume to this book, *An Introduction To Macrobiotics*, explains, in simple terms and examples, *why* it is that some foods are recommended while others are best avoided. In the macrobiotic view, foods are more than just a matter of vitamins, minerals, proteins, and carbohydrates; they profoundly affect us in other ways as well, to the degree that they can actually govern the way in which our physical and even our mental functions operate. The quality of our digestion, circulation, respiration, and nervous functions, to name only a few, can be heavily influenced by the *type* of foods we choose to consume. Knowing how this mechanism operates enables us to determine the state of our health, which profoundly influences the quality of our lives.

The following lists present a very condensed summary of those foods which are considered beneficial and wholesome from the macrobiotic perspective, and those which are not considered wholesome.

Whole grains and *vegetables* are the key foods in a macrobiotic diet. They have traditionally been the staple foods of people living in temperate climates, and have been extensively used in other climates as well. These two basic foods are supplemented by a wide range of soups, soyfoods, beans, fruits, nuts, seeds, fish, and sea greens. All of these foods can be prepared and incorporated in a variety of pleasing ways.

COMBINING FOODS

In the macrobiotic approach to nutrition, recommended foods are not eaten at random, such as only salad one day and lots of fruit the next. Such fluctuations in one's pattern of eating may cause highs and lows in mood, as well as functional disorders in the body. Rather, a macrobiotic diet considers not only *what* foods are eaten, but also the *way* in which they are consumed. They should be eaten in well-rounded, balanced meals—meals that can provide our bodies with the kind of complete nourishment that sustains good health.

The following pattern outlines the ideal proportion of grains, vegetables, and other whole foods appropriate for people living in a temperate zone climate. For those living in much colder or much warmer climates, these percentages would need to be adjusted slightly in accordance with temperature changes. For example, higher percentages of food from animal sources are recommended for people

FOODS RECOMMENDED

WHOLE GRAINS

Unrefined cereal grains, eaten either whole (brown rice, barley, millet, buckwheat, etc.) or as whole grain meal or flour in the form of pasta, noodles, and breads; and rolled, cracked, or steel-cut cereals.

VEGETABLES

Fresh vegetables (not canned or frozen), including leafy green and yellow vegetables, as well as root and stem vegetables, both cooked and raw.

PROTEIN - RICH FOODS

Foods high in vegetable proteins, in the form of beans, nuts, seeds, seitan (wheat meat), and soyfoods (tofu, tempeh, and miso), as well as fish and seafood.

SEA GREENS

Vegetables from the sea, which have traditionally been used in soups, salads, and side dishes (see Glossary).

SOUPS

Different varieties of freshly-made soups, such as vegetable, noodle, and bean soups—especially a nutritious soy-flavored soup called miso.

SWEETENERS

Fresh, dried, or cooked seasonal fruits and grain-malt sweeteners, such as barley malt and rice syrup.

BEVERAGES

Vegetable and fruit juices, mild herb teas, grain coffees, pure spring water, amasake, and various undyed teas, such as mu tea and kukicha.

FOODS *NOT* RECOMMENDED

REFINED GRAINS

Refined cereal grains, eaten whole (white rice, hominy, etc.) or as meal or flour, in the form of white-flour pasta and noodles or white bread and commercially-refined breakfast cereals.

VEGETABLES

Potatoes, tomatoes, eggplant, zucchini, and all vegetables belonging to the nightshade family, or those which are tropical in origin.

PROTEIN - RICH FOODS

Most animal products, such as red meat (beef, lamb, and pork), poultry (chicken, turkey, goose, and wild game), and eggs. All dairy foods, including cheese, butter, milk, yogurt, and ice cream.

ARTIFICIALLY - PROCESSED FOODS

Instant, canned, and frozen foods, and all foods processed with chemicals and additives, or artificial colorings or flavorings.

FATS & OILS

Lard and shortening, margarine, and refined vegetable oils.

SWEETENERS

Sugar (refined or brown), honey, molasses, corn syrup, chocolate, and all artificial sweeteners. Also, tropical and sub-tropical fruits, such as bananas, grapefruit, mangoes, oranges, papayas, figs, coconuts, and kiwi.

BEVERAGES

All artificial beverages, such as flavored instant drinks and soft drinks, as well as tropical or sub-tropical fruit juices. Also, alcoholic beverages, coffee, and commercially-dyed teas.

living in colder climates or higher altitudes, while higher percentages of vegetables and raw foods are more appropriate for those living in tropical climates.

The Basic Macrobiotic Diet

50% - 60% Whole Cereal Grains
20% - 30% Vegetables
5% - 10% Beans and Sea Greens
5% - 10% Soup (Miso, Vegetable, Fish, etc.)

Also included are seeds, fruits, nuts, and fish (based upon climate, individual activity, and need.)

Macrobiotic dietary recommendations are in accordance with many of the suggestions contained in the report prepared by the Select Committee on Nutrition and Human Needs, *Dietary Goals for the United States* (United States Senate, 1977). This is an excellent and highly recommended publication that is available from the U.S. Government Printing Office in Washington, D.C. *Dietary Goals for the United States* recommends that Americans:

- Increase their consumption of whole grains
- Increase their consumption of fruits and vegetables
- Decrease their consumption of meat
- Decrease their consumption of foods high in fat
- Decrease their consumption of sugar

It is interesting that these recommendations by the U.S. Government are closely aligned with basic macrobiotic dietary guidelines. These, in turn, were based on traditional dietary patterns around the world. This convergence of opinions—ancient and modern, Eastern and Western—seems to confirm a wide-ranging consensus on what our dietary pattern should be. Current research increasingly validates the traditional dietary pattern of many cultures; i.e., one that is high in unrefined carbohydrates and vegetables, and low in meat and fat. This diet appears to be the one most conducive to sound health and freedom from degenerative disease. These new findings, together with the rich store of dietary wisdom found in various traditional cultures, are beginning to solve many of the long-standing mysteries surrounding the subject of nutrition.

A Transitional Diet

Although most of us aspire to eat wholesome foods in ideal proportions, it is easy to forget to do so in the course of daily activities. Initially, it may seem that balancing the various types of foods in our diet to conform to recommended proportions requires more attention than we can give, without becoming overly preoccupied with our food.

Making the change to a macrobiotic diet requires a period of adjustment, especially if your previous diet consisted largely of meat, dairy products, or sugared foods. Therefore, just as you don't begin to jog by running in a marathon, or start out singing by attempting an opera, you should not expect to begin a macrobiotic diet overnight.

In view of these considerations, it can be helpful to begin with a *transitional* diet. Quite simply, this means a slow and sensible, step-by-step change from a diet centered around meat, dairy products, and sugar to one composed of grains, vegetables, and other natural, wholesome foods. A transitional diet gives your body the necessary time to adapt to new sources of nourishment, and affords you the opportunity to make gradual adjustments in your eating habits and patterns.

A transitional diet includes all of the foods which are recommended in a macrobiotic diet, as well as some of the more familiar foods you have been accustomed to eating. However, it does *not* include those foods considered least beneficial to our health, such as meat and sugar.

On the following chart (pages 10 and 11), the A section provides examples of the kinds of foods that are recommended for daily use; the B section gives examples of some transitional foods; and the C section gives examples of foods that are best avoided. B foods are those foods you may need to include in your diet for a period of time, *while slowly and steadily reducing the amount and frequency of their use.* C foods are those which are difficult, if not impossible, to balance in a long-term, healthful dietary plan.

Some people need a transitional diet for only a few months, while others may require it for as long as several years. There is really no set amount of time for using a transitional diet. In fact, some people may not need a transitional diet at all if their previous diet was relatively wholesome and balanced. We all have different eating habits. Some of us have developed relatively good eating habits in our formative years, but many of us have relied largely upon junk food, sweets, snacks, and convenience foods. Variations like these can make a big difference in how comfortable one is when beginning a macrobiotic diet.

A good way to begin the transition to a macrobiotic diet is by eating at least one complete macrobiotic meal every day. Keeping this as your main meal, you can use both other recommended foods and transitional foods according to your taste and need. With this one substantial and well-prepared meal as the center of your daily nourishment, you can gradually reduce and eliminate the transitional foods in the rest of your diet over a period of time.

The chart on pages 12 and 13 outlines a guide for a macrobiotic meal, which is suitable for those who are just beginning to shift from a diet based on meat, sugar, and dairy products to a more natural diet based on grains, vegetables, and other natural, whole, foods.

COOKING FOODS

The third important factor to consider in a macrobiotic diet is *how* foods should be cooked. Basically, this means learning the proper ways to prepare various kinds of whole foods, so that the meals you consume are neither too oily nor salty, neither undercooked nor overcooked, and contain a proper balance of ingredients.

Cooking is a skill that can actually alter the state of your health, for better or for worse. Little have we realized that this simple daily activity holds the key to our health and, as a result, our happiness in life. It is through this important but often underesti-

						ADUKI BEANS	
					BARLEY	BLACK BEANS	
					BREAD (SOURDOUGH)	CHICK	
				CARP	BROWN RICE	PEAS	CORN OIL
				CLAMS	BUCKWHEAT	KIDNEY	ALMONDS
				COD	CORN	BEANS	FILBERTS
				FLOUNDER	CORN MEAL	LENTILS	PEANUTS
				HADDOCK	COUSCOUS	LIMA	PECANS
				HALIBUT	CRACKED	BEANS	POPPY
				HERRING	WHEAT	NAVY	SEEDS
	BEEF			OYSTERS	MILLET	BEANS	PUMPKIN
	LAMB			RED	NOODLES	PINTO	SEEDS
	MUTTON			SNAPPER	OATS	BEANS	SAFFLOWER
	PORK			SCALLOPS	PASTA	SEITAN	OIL
	RABBIT	CHICKEN	BLUEFISH	SHRIMP	RYE	SOY BEANS	SESAME OIL
HEN'S	VEAL	DUCK	SALMON	SMELT	SWEET	SPLIT PEAS	SUNFLOWER
EGGS	WILD	GOOSE	SWORDFISH	SOLE	RICE	TEMPEH	SEEDS
CAVIAR	GAME	TURKEY	TUNA	TROUT	WHEAT	TOFU	WALNUTS
EGGS	MEAT	POULTRY	FISH & SEAFOOD	FISH & SEAFOOD	WHOLE GRAINS	PROTEINS	SEEDS, NUTS, & OILS

C   **B**   **A**

FOODS TO AVOID   TRANSITIONAL FOODS   RECOMMENDED FOODS

*It is suggested that transitional foods be eaten in smaller portions than usual, and that they be taken only as often as necessary instead of with every meal.

VEGETABLES	SEA GREENS	FRUITS	SWEETENERS	SWEETS & SNACKS	DAIRY FOODS	SWEETENERS	STIMULANTS
BROCCOLI							
CABBAGE							
CARROTS							
CAULIFLOWER							
CELERY							
COLLARDS				BANANAS			
CUCUMBERS				BRAZIL			
KALE				NUTS			
LEEKS		APPLES		CASHEWS			
LETTUCE		APRICOTS		COCONUT			
ONIONS		BLUEBERRIES		FIGS			
PARSLEY		CANTELOUPE		FRUIT			
PARSNIPS		CHERRIES		JUICES			
PEAS	AGAR	CHESTNUTS		GRAPEFRUIT			
RADISHES	AGAR	GRAPES		LEMONS			
SCALLIONS	ARAME	PEACHES		MAPLE	BUTTER	ARTIFICIAL	
SQUASH	DULSE	PEARS	APPLE	SYRUP	CHEESE	SWEETENERS	
BEANS	HIZIKI	PLUMS	BUTTER	OLIVES	CREAM	CHOCOLATE	
STRING	KELP	RAISINS	BARLEY	ORANGES	ICE	CORN SYRUP	
SWISS CHARD	KOMBU	RASPBERRIES	MALT	PAPAYAS	CREAM	HONEY	ALCOHOL
TURNIPS	NORI	STRAWBERRIES	FRUIT JUICE	VEGETABLE	MILK	MOLASSES	DRUGS
WATERCRESS	WAKAME	WATERMELON	RICE SYRUP	JUICES	YOGURT	SUGAR	SPICES

A

RECOMMENDED FOODS

B

TRANSITIONAL FOODS

C

FOODS TO AVOID

*Due to space limitations, this chart does not give a complete listing of all the foods that may be included in the macrobiotic diet. Rather, it gives a general indication of foods recommended for use in temperate zone climates.

WHOLE GRAINS

Whole grains & foods made from whole grain flour and meal, including bread, pasta and noodles, cracked wheat, corn meal, etc.

FRESH VEGETABLES

Freshly-cooked vegetables, including a daily variety of root and stem vegetables and leafy greens.

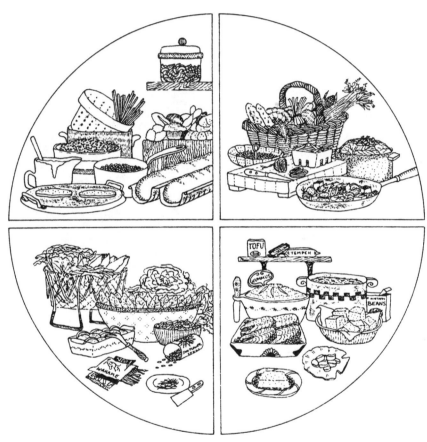

COMBINATION DISHES

Changing combinations of sea vegetables, fresh salads, pickles, seeds, and nuts.

PROTEIN - RICH FOODS

Tempeh (soy meat), tofu (soy cheese), seitan (wheat meat), beans, & occasionally fish.

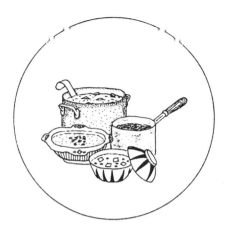

SOUPS

A variety of freshly-made soups containing beans, grains, sea greens, vegetables, and miso or tamari soy sauce for seasoning.

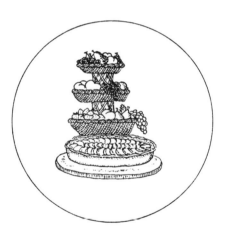

DESSERTS

Fresh fruits; naturally-sweetened desserts, such as puddings, pies, kanten-gelatins, or cakes sweetened with malt syrup.

This chart shows only a general guideline for beginning a macrobiotic diet. Initially, the proportion of grains, vegetables, proteins, and other foods consumed may be according to individual taste, but gradually *whole grains* should play a central role in one's diet, followed by *vegetables, proteins*, and *combination foods*, as outlined in the standard macrobiotic diet. More information on the standard macrobiotic diet may be found in *The Macrobiotic Way*, by Michio Kushi, and in other publications listed in Appendix C.

mated art that we control what we absorb into our being. Therefore, it is important to learn the art of cooking *attentively* and to practice it well, for there is much more to preparing meals than just creating pleasant tastes. Learning how to prepare food in a healthful, yet still delicious, manner is an essential step on the road to health and longevity.

Cooking will be discussed in more detail in Chapter 5.

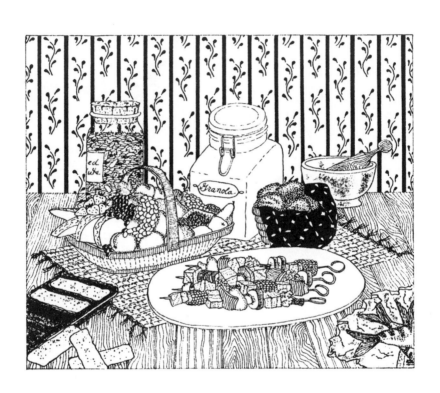

2

The Period of Adjustment

In one sense, it is not at all difficult to switch to a better diet, since natural foods, when properly prepared, can be quite delicious. But it *can* be somewhat difficult to keep from eating bad foods. When we begin to decrease our intake of certain foods that we would like to give up, we often find that many of them are almost *addictive*. We all know the cravings a "junk food junkie" has for potato chips, soda, hamburgers, ice cream, or candy bars.

Giving up unwholesome foods is no different from giving up cigarettes, coffee, or any other substance to which we have long been accustomed. A few of us may be able to relinquish our ice cream cones, hot dogs, or other favorites all at once, but most of us find this to be too much of a shock to our systems. Although intellectually we can understand the importance of eating well and can easily decide to change our eating habits, we must realize that our bodies change more slowly than our thought processes do, at rhythms inherent to a physical, organic process. Therefore, it is usually wise to proceed gradually and to give our bodies the time they need to adapt to more wholesome sources of nourishment.

EXAMINING OLD HABITS

Regardless of the kind of diet one may adopt, experience has shown that sharp reactions are likely to occur after an enforced period of quick change. In other words, if we try too hard, or if we are too strict with ourselves in the beginning, we may encounter various problems (such as uncontrollable food binges) that leave us feeling discouraged. Binges may also result in response to extreme fluctuations in the glucose level of the blood. You can prevent these by being sensitive to your body's needs and by learning the effects of various foods on your body (see Appendix C). Binges are less likely to occur if you make sure you include a sufficient *variety* of grains, beans, vegetables, sea greens, soups, and seeds in your diet, and vary the ways in which you prepare them.

If you experience frequent food binges, you may need to put more thought and effort into the preparation of your meals. You may find that you are too busy (or unwilling) to cook proper meals. Any of these problems can lead to an irregular pattern of eating and have undesirable effects on your health. But even rigid or lazy attitudes can be changed, in time, into a more relaxed and responsible view. In fact, such self-inflicted difficulties eventually force us to retrace our steps and begin again in a more sensible way.

Setting a rigid goal for yourself may only set you up for failure. Instead, be realistic about where you happen to be in the process of changing your diet. Remember that your food preferences—even your sense of taste—will change and improve with the passage of time, and you will be able to discern a clear evolution in your eating habits. But this takes patience and the essential factor of time. (This is no excuse, however, for unnecessary self-indulgence.)

Eventually, you must find the right balance for yourself. This should be somewhere between being overly relaxed about your diet, on the one hand, and overly watchful, on the other.

After shedding some unwanted pounds, suffering from fewer colds and headaches, and sporting a clearer complexion and a more positive attitude, you will find that the benefits of natural foods make it easier to skip the unwholesome ones and reach for a healthier choice. Few people return to their old habits once they have seen for themselves the effect of various foods on their health, and once they have begun to experience the sense of well-being that accompanies a macrobiotic, whole foods diet.

CHANGING HABITS

The first step towards improving your diet is to eliminate those foods that are the most extreme and the most harmful in your diet, such as meat and sugar. Next, begin to include whole grain cereals and naturally-leavened breads, and reduce your intake of such dairy products as ice cream and cheese. Begin to replace frozen foods and canned goods with fresh foods. Also, become acquainted with various soyfoods and sweeteners made from malted grains, such as barley-malt syrup and rice syrup. One by one, try different ways of cooking whole grains and soyfoods. Get to know the many different types—and tastes— of natural foods.

At first, it may be difficult to pass up a slice of pizza, an ice cream sundae, or any number of other tempting but unwholesome foods. In fact, it would be unusual if you did *not* experience a desire for such foods, just as it would be unusual for a cigarette smoker not to experience a craving for nicotine when attempting to give up smoking. Therefore, when cravings for sugar, meat, or dairy foods do arise, it helps to replace them with more wholesome foods of a *similar type*.

For example, if you usually have donuts or sweet rolls for breakfast, try substituting whole wheat muffins or donuts made with a more wholesome sweetener such as barley-malt or rice syrup. If it is meat, eggs, or cheese you crave, replace them with other foods that are rich in protein and natural oils— such as fish or seafood, soyfoods, beans, and nuts. A variety of cheese substitutes can be made with tofu; let your macrobiotic cookbook be your guide. If a hamburger is the food you long for, you may want to experiment with the various brands of tofu burgers, tempeh burgers, or "veggie-burgers" available at your natural foods store. You'll also find there a variety of natural sweets and snacks, from candy to corn chips. You may find these items useful in your transition from a diet of highly-processed and chemicalized foods to one that is more wholesome. But remember that ready-made foods, no matter how natural the ingredients, are no substitute for home-cooked meals.

The goal is not to replace your favorite meat or cheese dish with your favorite health-burger, but to deal with your cravings in a sensible way. By introducing yourself to new and appropriate foods, you will increase your range of wholesome choices that will not only please your palate but satisfy your cravings as well.

As we begin to eat more wholesome foods, our bodies begin to cleanse themselves internally. This process sometimes includes the discharge of toxins and deposits of fat and mucous that have been built up over the years from a diet containing excessive amounts of saturated fats, sugars, and chemicals.

Therefore, like a good exercise program, a good diet is something that is best built up over a period of months. Each adjustment will increase your capacity to make further improvements in your health, create a deeper understanding of how you are affected by your diet, and promote a greater enjoyment and appreciation of foods as well.

Just as winter changes into summer through the transition state of spring, the transition from a diet centered around meat, dairy, and sugar products to a diet centered around grains and vegetables takes place during a kind of "spring," as the two diets begin to merge for a while.

EXAMINING PATTERNS

One way to ease this period of adjustment is to duplicate one's previous food patterns for a while, only using better-quality ingredients. For example, if you tend to eat salad quite regularly, continue to have it, but begin using a better-quality salad dressing (one without artificial flavorings, colorings, sugar, etc.). You might also eliminate less beneficial ingredients, such as tomatoes or mayonnaise.

If you have a strong sweet tooth, use naturally-sweetened desserts as a more wholesome alternative, and keep favorite fruits in stock as well. If you are in the habit of snacking, don't expect to eliminate this habit overnight, either. Instead, provide yourself with better-quality, natural snacks, of which there is a plentiful variety (corn chips, rice cakes, fresh fruits, granola, dried fruits, roasted nuts, pickles, olives, whole grain crackers, and various dips, spreads, and jams). Whatever your habits are, it helps to take note of them, and to follow the same general dietary pattern for a while, gradually introducing new and more healthy foods into your diet. Poor eating habits can't be changed overnight, but with time and patience, you and your family can eventually establish a better way of eating.

FRIENDS AND FAMILY

Family members and friends are likely to react to your new diet in a variety of ways. At least one person you know will probably ruffle your feathers with a few wry comments about your new foods, while others may instantly credit you with the title of nutrition expert and begin to question you about everything from asparagus to zucchini. Eating foods that are different does necessitate a sharpening of your social skills. At least you won't be found lacking in lively conversation, since nearly everyone these days is interested in learning more about the relationship between diet and health.

Should any of your friends or relatives look askance at your new diet, you can put them at ease by resisting the temptation to make a speech about the importance of good nutrition. Just because dietary awareness has become a part of *your* life, don't assume that friends and relatives will automatically share your enthusiasm.

Nevertheless, it is only natural to want the people you care about to eat foods that are good for them, rather than those which may be harmful. This is especially true with regard to members of your immediate family—your spouse, your parents, and your children. But this desire is not always easily fulfilled. In matters of diet, people tend to get set in their ways rather early in life. Still, people can and do change sometimes, and you may find that eventually your influence will be important to those around you. But when first acquainting your family with foods that are unfamiliar to them, remember that a macrobiotic diet usually requires a period of adjustment. So be sure to allow for this when trying to raise their awareness concerning matters of diet.

Avoid introducing them to too many new foods at once. Quite naturally, they would be disconcerted upon finding the table bereft of all familiar foods, and replaced by those which are new and different. Keep this in mind, and prepare foods that are somewhat similar in taste, texture, and appearance to those they usually eat. Try serving soyburgers, bean tacos, soy-cheese spreads, whole grain pasta, fruit gelatins, whole wheat rolls, noodle soup, and other familiar foods that can be made with natural ingredients.

Meanwhile, it helps to begin using the best quality foods that you can possibly find. Substitute raw milk for regular milk, unsweetened jam for sugar-sweetened jam, dried or fresh fruits and vegetables for canned and frozen ones, unleavened and sourdough breads for yeasted ones, and so on. Although you should avoid eliminating all your former foods at once, do begin to reduce the quantity and frequency with which you take them.

In time, these changes can work wonders, as you make gradual refinements in your family's diet, and learn to prepare meals that both meet their needs and protect their health. Once they have become more familiar with wholesome foods, their tastes are likely to change, and they will begin to prefer what is good for them. This depends largely on your skill as a cook, however, and just as importantly on your *diplomacy.*

When it comes to adopting a better diet and a healthier lifestyle, your spouse is likely to be the most important person involved. Often, one partner takes the lead in introducing the rest of the family to a more natural diet. But the transition works best when couples learn about whole, natural foods together.

Few couples can successfully cope with two kinds of diets in one household, although some do, in fact, manage this. You can help your spouse to better understand your new food preferences by having a serious discussion with him or her, clearly stating your reasons why a whole foods diet is important to you. Without insistence or pressure, encourage your mate to try some natural foods. If you meet with disinterest, being patient will help.

Don't isolate yourself, though. Share dinners and discussions with friends or other groups. Attend whole foods workshops, lectures, or classes in your area. This will not only help you to learn more, but will also enable you to establish the base of support necessary for your sense of well-being. Get to know the natural food stores in your area. You may find a neighbor, a gardener, a health professional, or simply a new friend with a perspective on diet similar to yours.

Don't separate yourself from other people because of your food preferences. You can enjoy dining out with friends even though the menu has little to offer in the way of natural foods. There is no reason why you shouldn't enjoy good company just because you eat differently. On such occasions, make wise choices from the fare that is offered, taking some tips from those offered in the next chapter. Likewise, at a party, nursing a glass of mineral water, fruit juice, or beer will alleviate any discomfort you or your hosts might feel, were you to flatly reject their hospitality.

Parents respond quite differently to changes in their children's diets. Some parents are tolerant of their children's 'fads,' while others fret. Some are wonderfully supportive and broad-minded. If your parents seem to be worried about your new diet, have a talk with them about the nutritional soundness of a macrobiotic diet. The initial weight loss experienced by most people when beginning a macrobiotic diet is only the trimming of excess—unless you are eating inadequate meals—but this can be alarming to parents who tend to equate "healthy" with "plump." Unless you've been eating incorrectly, you should not experience drastic weight loss, although this may happen if you were extremely overweight to begin with.

Put your parents at ease, when visiting them, by eating whatever is healthiest amongst their fare— vegetables, soups, salads, breads, fish dishes, hot cereals, and so on. In this way, they won't feel excluded or separated from your life. Food is an important physical and psychological bond between people, so refrain from criticizing their way of eating. If you think they might be interested, give them a few whole grain recipes for whole wheat bread or some other dish you think they might enjoy. After a while, when they see that your diet is a serious choice rather than a passing fad, they may begin to cook fish instead of meat when you join them for dinner, and offer you fresh fruit instead of cake for dessert.

Cooking dinner for *them*, occasionally, can help your parents to see your side of things, too. You'll not only have an opportunity to show off your culinary talents, but you'll also be giving your parents a chance to experience the great variety, and even elegance, of macrobiotic foods. Take these opportunities to offset any notion they may have that a macrobiotic diet is all carrots and brown rice. Prepare apple pie, corn chowder, fish kebabs, fresh salads, baked beans, or other familiar foods, using wholesome ingredients. In time, as you share your food, and they see how much you value good nutrition, you'll feel better knowing that your parents may be keeping a more watchful eye on what they eat, too.

If you are a parent, however, *your* children are another matter. If you help them to understand little by little, children can sometimes be surprisingly cooperative about changing to a better diet. Begin by making small changes, such as switching to a natural type of peanut butter without sugar or chemicals, an unsweetened jelly, granola or muesli cereals, pure fruit juices, and whole grain breads and muffins. If you *add* some healthy foods before subtracting unhealthy ones, you are more likely to get a better response. Good cooking is more effective than talking, at first. Give your children tasty, wholesome meals *without* a lecture. Answer their questions, but avoid preaching. They will learn better habits little by little, as you make further improvements and adjustments in their diets. Any insistence on your part, or an abrupt change in their diets, is likely to result in an outright rejection of natural foods and new ideas.

Of course, one must be careful with children, since they are too young to be responsible for their own health. Too much leniency with candy, sugar, soda, and so on can be very harmful for them. But being too strict, at the outset, can alienate them permanently from the more healthful foods you would like them to enjoy. It becomes, therefore, a matter of your own judgment, exercised daily, to discern when to be lenient and when to be firm and offer a more healthful alternative. Best of all is to simply set a good example by preparing delicious, satisfying meals—every day—using natural whole foods.

Depending upon the willingness and openness of your spouse—if you are married—and upon the attitudes of your children—if you are a parent—it may take either a very short or a very long time to change your home into a healthier one. But by placing emphasis on introducing beneficial foods, rather than on eliminating detrimental ones, you can steer your family's diet in a positive direction during this time of transition. Avoid nagging them about their eating habits. Every individual has a choice, and this choice should be respected.

Take a cue from Mother Nature and be patient. As She well knows, evolution takes a little time. Spare your family and friends the ordeal of having to live with a zealot, but retain your commitment to a healthful diet. Every year, thousands of individuals make this same adjustment, gradually changing their family's health for the better, and day-by-day improving the quality of their lives.

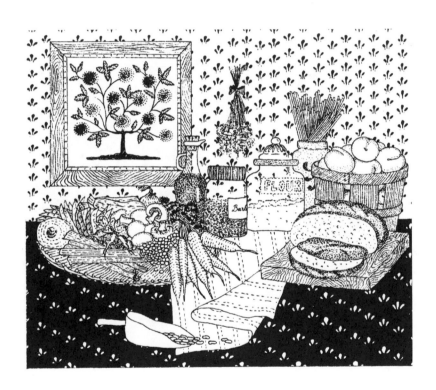

3

Breakfast, Lunch, & Dinner

BREAKFAST

Without eggs, bacon, orange juice, and milk, most people wonder what's left to eat for breakfast, especially when they don't have much time to cook in the morning. As shown in the last chapter, it helps to take note of your former breakfast habits and to initially follow this same pattern.

If you are accustomed to eating hot or cold cereals, for example, try switching to an unsweetened, *whole grain* cereal. Instead of milk, try amasake, a naturally-sweetened 'cream' which is made from whole grains. If you are in the habit of having pancakes with syrup, try whole wheat sourdough pancakes or waffles, with applesauce or fruit puree. Ham and eggs? Try soy "sausage" and scrambled tofu with whole wheat English muffins or toast.

Unfortunately, most of the breakfast foods we eat today are sweet, and it's best not to overindulge in sweets, even when they are made from good-quality ingredients. You can always satisfy your sweet tooth with a more wholesome sweet, instead of a sugary donut. Many natural foods cookbooks offer excellent recipes for breakfast foods of all kinds. Also, you might want to check your natural foods store for a selection of wholesome breakfast rolls and cereals which may not be available in bakeries and supermarkets.

Some people enjoy a full and varied breakfast, while others prefer a light and simple one. Still others would rather skip breakfast altogether. The important point is to have at least two hearty and well-balanced meals every day. A scanty breakfast is not harmful, provided that lunch and dinner are ample and nutritious. But a light breakfast *and* a light lunch will probably induce impulsive snacking on cookies, crackers, or whatever else is close at hand. This will only reinforce poor eating habits and eventually lead to an anemic condition. So make up for a light breakfast with a good, hearty lunch. If it is a light lunch you prefer, then start the day with a substantial and varied breakfast.

Most growing children enjoy and *need* a hot breakfast—one that is not too sweet and that is high in nutrition. In addition, if you have a high-energy, demanding job, it is best to begin the day with a hearty breakfast. This will provide you with the energy you will need all morning.

LUNCH

Maintaining a wholesome diet *can* present a problem on occasion. For example, it may be difficult to find an acceptable restaurant to eat in. When the local burger stop is no longer an option—nor the neighborhood deli, pizza place, or chicken chain—where do you go when you want a wholesome lunch away from the office or home? Most restaurants offer only a chemical feast—monosodium glutamate, artificial colorings, flavorings, and preservatives—and a menu consisting mostly of meat, dairy products, and sugary desserts.

As surrounded as we are by restaurants these days, there are really very few places that offer a wholesome meal. The coffee shop down the street may serve fish, but its appearance and flavor are likely to be altered to a point beyond recognition. The accompanying pale salad is often sprayed with chemicals to keep the lettuce from wilting during its long hours on the salad bar, and the bread is not what one would readily call the staff of life, but something more akin to sponge. Practically everything you can possibly order has been liberally doused with chemicals and preservatives. Until these establishments begin to improve the quality of their fare, they are not a healthful option. Where, then, is a good meal to be found? Clearly we are obliged to consider more carefully where to dine.

In large cities there is often an abundance of ethnic restaurants, where the meals are likely to bear more resemblance to real food. By choosing carefully from their menus, it is often possible to put together a passable meal.

For instance, a few good dishes can be found in Chinese restaurants, although Chinese chefs have the unfortunate habit of lacing everything with monosodium glutamate or lard. In some of the better Chinese restaurants, however, one can often persuade the cook to prepare a stir-fried vegetable, rice, or fish dish that is free of these two ingredients. (In many ethnic restaurants, it is necessary to request that only vegetable oil be used in preparing your food, rather than butter or lard.)

Mexican restaurants offer rice, beans, salad, tortillas, and a few other dishes made without meat, such as meatless tostadas, tamales, and burritos. Almost everything else, however, is inundated with cheese. While this range of choices is somewhat limited, it can still serve as an occasional alternative.

Greek, Israeli, and Middle Eastern restaurants offer several vegetarian items such as falafels (chick-pea croquettes), hummus (chick-pea spread), pita bread, olives, salad, and some good side dishes, such as meatless stuffed grape leaves. Indian restaurants usually serve a good lentil dish, called *dahl*, along with chapatis or puri (traditional unleavened breads), a vegetarian soup, as well as vegetables and salad.

Japanese restaurants offer eggless noodles, *tempura* (deep-fried vegetables or fish), *sushi* (bite-sized rounds of rice and fish or rice and vegetables), and salad or boiled greens. Check out other specialties, too, such as sea greens or tofu dishes, but inquire about the use of monosodium glutamate and sugar in any item you order. In Vietnamese, Thai, and Indonesian restaurants, the chef will often prepare a fresh vegetable or fish dish, served over rice.

Continental restaurants provide highly limited choices unless, of course, you are at one of the very best, in which case you may be able to order a beautiful platter of perfectly-cooked vegetables prepared by a chef who *understands* vegetable cookery. Otherwise, a broiled or grilled fish and a green salad are your best bet.

Italian restaurants in America do not usually present the more refined side of Italian cooking, which has a simplicity and lightness that the cheese-laden American versions altogether miss. But should you happen to know of a good one, you may be able to obtain either an excellent minestrone soup or pasta dish, as well as freshly-cooked vegetables and fruit. If you are fortunate enough to live or work near a natural foods restaurant, the menu is likely to offer several excellent choices. While most natural foods restaurants are not yet bastions of haute cuisine, at least these establishments are on the right track. All too often, however, the majority of entrees are camouflaged by a thick coating of melted cheese or an excess of spices. (A good cook can bring out the flavor of foods without the use of MSG, spices, cheese, or heavy sauces).

After playing around with the above alternatives for a while, one usually decides to bring lunch from home. Perhaps the easiest wholesome lunch you can make is a thermos of hot soup (vegetable, miso, barley, macaroni, or chowder) and a sandwich (sprout, hummus, wheat meat, fried tempeh, or falafel, to name a few). Add vegetables, salad, or fresh fruit according to season, and you have a fairly simple, yet nourishing, midday meal. Homemade lunches are usually the most healthful and are well worth the effort it takes to prepare them.

School children sometimes face the problem of classmate disapproval of foods that "look different." This can turn your children against the foods you would like them to eat. Therefore, it's best to prepare lunches which at least look like the lunches brought by their classmates. This can be done using a variety of wholesome soups, sandwiches, fruits, and vegetables.

If your children attend a school with a cafeteria, you may want to ask the administrators to introduce some better foods into the menu. Many parents have convinced administrators and cafeteria managers to serve more natural foods and to cut back on artificial snacks and sweets. This influence is being felt from California to Massachusetts, and many schools have already begun to include natural foods in their cafeteria menus.

DINNER

It doesn't take a connoisseur to realize that family dining is quickly becoming a lost art. Some years ago, family meals began with a prayer of thanks, followed by a ladeling of the soup, after which everyone was ready to savor both the food and the conversation. Today, however, we no longer seem to observe the simple courtesies that once graced our meals. In fact, in homes and restaurants across the nation, it is not uncommon for people to wolf down their food and run from the table—more or less "feed" than dine as it were. Needless to say, consuming food in this fashion is harmful to our digestion and has a dampening effect on the pleasures of conversation and conviviality as well.

It is best to chew our food well, and eat in an unhurried and pleasant atmosphere. Therefore, it is well worth investing a little time and energy in creating an enjoyable and relaxed environment. Even small touches, such as flowers and a tablecloth, can improve the ambiance of a room in subtle ways and elevate the act of eating to the art of dining. Also, saying a prayer of thanks before meals helps to create a peaceful atmosphere and sets the tone for gentle conversation.

By practicing poor eating habits, several things can happen. Chewing poorly or eating too fast interferes with our ability to assimilate nutrients, while overeating or constant snacking results in bloating and indigestion. By reminding ourselves to chew well, we can assist our bodies in the process of digestion. With a little effort, we can begin to reverse our tendency to "eat-and-run." This requires the commitment of a little extra time and attention when preparing and enjoying wholesome meals.

The following menus provide only a small sample of the unlimited ways of preparing breakfast, lunch, and dinner using recommended foods. Remember that macrobiotic dinners can be either plain and simple or elaborate and fancy, depending on the occasion. They can be easily adapted for casual backyard gatherings or for such special events as weddings and holiday feasts. Further ideas for interesting menus can be found in macrobiotic cookbooks, a number of which are now available at most bookstores and natural foods stores.

SAMPLE TRANSITION MENUS

	Sunday	Monday	Tuesday
BREAKFAST	Whole grain waffles with applesauce Grain coffee	Seven-grain hot cereal Corn muffins Amasake	Whole grain pancakes with jelly Fried tempeh sausage Herb tea
LUNCH	Onion soup Falafel sandwich in whole wheat pita bread with tahini dressing Mixed vegetable Amasake fruit shake	Vegetable noodle soup Tempeh sandwich Green vegetable Fresh fruit cup	Lentil soup Wheat meat sandwich with lettuce & mustard Green vegetable
DINNER	Fresh corn soup Millet croquettes Baked halibut Green salad Cherry turnover	Miso soup Brown rice pilaf Wheat meat–and–vegetable stew Mixed salad	Noodles in vegetable broth Batter - fried fish & vegetables Sea greens with sesame seeds Cucumber salad Fruit gelatin (kanten)

SAMPLE TRANSITION MENUS

Wednesday	Thursday	Friday	Saturday
Whole wheat croissant	Whole grain cold cereal with amasake	Scrambled tofu with whole wheat English muffins	Whole wheat blueberry muffins
Hot sesame-oat cereal with amasake	Hot corn bread		Oatmeal
Split-pea soup	Barley vegetable soup	Fresh fruit cup	Sliced strawberries
Soyburger with pickles on whole wheat roll	Hummus (chick-pea spread) with whole wheat pita bread & olives	Miso soup	Macaroni vegetable soup
Coleslaw		Pasta salad	Fried fish fillet
Fruit tart	Mixed salad	Roasted nuts	Green vegetable
			Hot cider
Fish chowder	Minestrone soup	Vegetable soup	Squash soup
Wheat pilaf	Brown rice	Stir-fried vegetables and shrimp over long-grain brown rice	Pinto beans with carrots & onions
Tempeh with onion gravy	Broiled fillet of sole with lemon		Corn tortillas
Steamed vegetables	Baked squash	Green salad	Deep-fried onion rings
Mixed salad with sea greens	Steamed broccoli	Apple pie	Mixed salad
	Tahini custard		

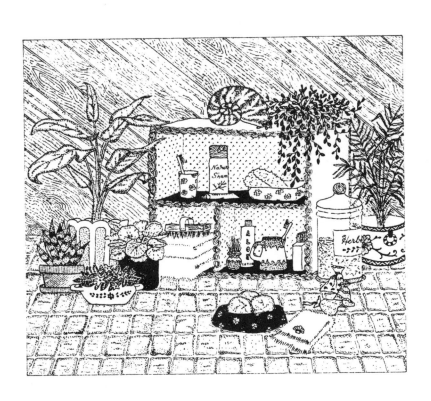

4

Helpful Suggestions

NATURAL LIVING

In addition to dietary recommendations, a macrobiotic health care program also encompasses lifestyle changes. The following suggestions can help you to create a more natural way of life and a healthier home environment. In a world that is becoming increasingly artificial and polluted, these suggestions are all the more useful.

Natural Fiber Clothing

Synthetic materials trap perspiration and body toxins. Therefore, it's best not to encase your body in such artificial substances as nylon, polyester, or acrylic all day. Natural fibers allow your skin to "breathe" more effectively. Thus, natural materials—such as cotton and linen—are not only more comfortable, but they are also better for your health. Wool and silk are also good choices, but cotton is the best material to wear directly next to your skin. Pure cotton is also ideal for sheets. Finally, it is best to choose natural fibers such as cotton, wool, and silk for bed covers, blankets, and comforters.

Natural Soaps and Cosmetics

It makes no more sense to rub chemicals on your body than it does to put them in your food. You can avoid this problem by using shampoos, soaps, and cosmetics made from natural herbs, roots, and minerals, and which are free from the chemical additives so widely used in toiletries today.

Another reason for avoiding these chemicalized soaps and cosmetics is the sad fact that some seventy million animals die each year in American laboratories. Many of these animals are used to test everyday products that we use in our homes, from hairsprays to deodorants. In most cases, these tests involve a prolonged ordeal of cruel and inhumane torture. Such testing is entirely unnecesssary for the production or development of safe toiletries, and companies which support such testing should not be patronized.

One organization which is doing something to monitor and change this situation is *Beauty Without Cruelty* (175 West 12th St., Suite 166, New York, NY 10011). By sending them a self-addressed, stamped envelope, you can obtain a list of those soap and cosmetic companies that do *not* utilize cruel tests in creating their products. These lists are available for countries other than the United States as well. Many of these brands can be found in most natural foods stores.

Exercise

Everyone knows that exercise is important in order to maintain good health. It is, however, easy to put off, or to forget about altogether, unless it is regularly scheduled. Some people enjoy very active exercise, like cycling, jogging, racquetball, or team sports. Others favor quiet, meditative exercise, like yoga or walking. Some people simply prefer housework, yardwork, or gardening. But some form of exercise should be performed every day, not only for the physical conditioning and flexibility it provides but also for mental relaxation. This need not be an exhausting or demanding regimen. It should, however, be a regular habit that is practiced consistently. A regular routine of brisk walking, jogging, or indoor exercise once a day will make a big difference in the quality of your digestion, circulation, and respiration.

Green Plants

The beauty of green plants can add greatly to the atmosphere of your home or office. But these graceful decorations do more than simply beautify your surroundings—they also enrich the air with oxygen. Adding some large green plants to your home will not only freshen the atmosphere, but will add a more natural note to the environment.

Recent NASA experiments have shown that houseplants remove common indoor air pollutants such as carbon monoxide, nitrogen dioxide, and formaldehyde. Three or four plants in a 12′ x 15′ room will continuously freshen and filter the air.

Electrical Appliances

Microwave ovens, television sets, and a host of other electrical appliances can alter the atmosphere of our homes in subtle ways. By altering the ratio of positively-charged and negatively-charged ions in the air, these devices can produce a less natural atmosphere. Therefore, it is wise to avoid excessive use of electrical appliances and such items as electric blankets. Microwave devices, television sets, and computer terminals can also be sources of low-level radiation, and their use should be minimized as much as possible.

In addition, using an electrical appliance to cook your food makes it difficult to control the subtle changes in temperature so essential to fine cooking. Electricity (high-wattage electrical energy) can also affect the quality of your food. Switching to a gas stove will allow you to cook in a more natural way, using fire.

Sleeping

As a general rule, it is best to follow the natural cycle of the sun—going to sleep early, rising early, and so on. Frequently staying up past midnight, or lounging in bed until noon, disrupts our natural rhythm and our individual harmony with the order of the day.

It is also important to allow about three hours between your last meal and going to sleep. Like the rest of your body, the stomach and intestines also need rest. But if you eat right before going to sleep, your digestive organs cannot fully rest or function properly. This causes stagnation in your digestive tract, and may contribute to such problems as obesity, increased appetite, or a tired, sluggish feeling in the morning.

Spring Water

The kind of water that you use for cooking and drinking is also very important. In most cities and towns, the tap water has been treated with numerous chemicals that not only affect the taste of the water (and, as a result, the taste of the foods you cook) but also the quality and content of what you put into your body. Fortunately, in most cities there are spring water companies that will deliver 5-gallon bottles of pure spring or well water for a relatively low cost. Water is an important component of a good diet and one which deserves a few moments of your time to locate a good source. Avoid using distilled water, however, which has been sterilized and is therefore a dead and lifeless form of this all-important substance.

Chewing

Chewing is an important step in the digestive process, for digestion actually begins *in the mouth* with enzymes from our saliva. Chewing also helps our bodies to assimilate food nutrients by grinding them into smaller particles and transforming them into a more liquid state. So in order to fully benefit from a whole foods diet, thorough chewing is necessary.

Although chewing food well is not difficult, it is easy to forget this in the course of our daily activities. Try chewing very well for one or two days, and you will immediately see for yourself what a big difference it can make in the way you feel. Remind yourself before every meal to slow down and chew. You'll digest your food better, and eat less, too.

WHERE TO SHOP

Natural foods from reputable distributors are now available in most cities and many smaller towns as well. Nearly every major city has several natural foods stores, where you can purchase whole grains, dried beans, nuts, seeds, sea greens, whole grain sourdough bread, expeller-pressed vegetable oil, unrefined sea salt, and all the basic staples you need. Though we live in an age where the basics of natural nutrition are not common knowledge, natural foods *are* becoming more popular every year. If this trend continues, natural foods will soon be available everywhere.

Beware, however, of health food stores which are only enlarged "pill boxes," offering you vitamins, supplements, and protein powders but very little real food. Many of the so-called "natural" products offered in such places—like brown sugar cookies and candy bars made with honey—are no better than supermarket fare. Such places will encourage you to overindulge in pills and supplements. Steer clear of them.

If there is no natural foods store in your area, try shopping by mail—at least for basic items. Many natural foods distributors will send you a catalog of the foods they ship, which will include weights, prices, and shipping costs. You can also write directly to natural foods processors, who can refer you to the nearest retail outlet or mail order company that handles their products. Mail order purchasing is especially useful for those living in rural areas, where—ironically—there are few sources of natural whole foods.

(See Appendix D for a listing of some major mail-order companies which carry a good selection of natural foods.)

Your next choice is a supermarket or, better yet, a farmer's market. Some supermarkets have installed natural foods sections in recent years, where you will find at least some of the things you need. But some of the so-called "natural" foods recently marketed by major companies may not be as natural as they seem. They often contain questionable ingredients, so check all packages carefully for the list of ingredients. In their other departments, supermarkets also have some whole grains, whole grain flours and meal, hot cereals, and several kinds of dried beans. Of course, you'll also find fresh vegetables and fruits and perhaps some nuts, seeds, or dried fruits.

When purchasing any macrobiotic product, be aware that certain so-called macrobiotic foods are not really of macrobiotic quality. Though some of the recently-established natural foods companies have every intention of providing their customers with good quality foods, they do not always have the necessary depth of understanding concerning the finer points of macrobiotic nutrition. As a result, some of the ways they process their products, some of the ingredients they use, and some of the combinations they create—while not particularly harmful—arc not particularly healthful, either. Many of them definitely do *not* contribute to a healing process. Your best protection against being misled by these well-intentioned natural foods or "macrobiotic" companies that may not be providing a really wholesome product is to be *informed*. The more you know about macrobiotic nutrition, the more you will be able to choose the foods you eat with care and understanding. As you become more educated and experienced with regard to the true macrobiotic quality of natural whole foods, insist on top quality and proper processing from your regional suppliers of whole foods—such as mochi, amasake, and miso, or prepared foods from the re-frigerator-section of your natural foods store—and do not be duped by packaging or the words "natural" or "macrobiotic quality." Remember, too, that natural frozen desserts can be helpful temporarily in a transitional diet as a substitute for ice cream, but should eventually be discontinued in favor of more healthful desserts.

If you are fortunate enough to have a good natural foods store in your area, you may want to make a copy of the shopping list at the back of this book to use as a shopping aid, until shopping natural comes "naturally."

Remember that *natural foods* contain no preservatives or additives to control appearance, texture, or shelf-life. For instance, in a jar of natural peanut butter, the oil will separate and rise to the top if it is not stirred for a period of time. This is because no additive has been used to keep the oil from separating. Such minor points should be of little importance to anyone interested in consuming foods that are uncontaminated with chemicals and additives.

Whole foods are foods in which no edible part of the natural grain, bean, seed, nut, fruit, or vegetable has been removed. Furthermore, in macrobiotic cooking, the method of cooking grains and beans whole is generally preferred to cracking, crushing, or grinding them before they are cooked. In preparing vegetables, the whole plant is used, including all edible roots, leaves, skins, cores, or stems.

Eating macrobiotically naturally encourages the use of foods that are organically grown, or foods that are grown without the use of artificial, chemical pesticides and herbicides. A system of farming that is based on the use of harmful chemicals is self-defeating to the purpose of providing sound human nourishment for generations far into the future—therefore, the macrobiotic approach to nutrition endorses organic farming as a more sustainable system of agriculture. The regeneration of our agricultural lands and waters is now of major, critical importance—both to the public's health and to future generations. We can help contribute to a healthier future by patronizing farmers and gardeners who practice this wiser, more natural system of organic agriculture.

POINTS TO REMEMBER

Salt

Salt addicts can be every bit as hooked as sugar addicts. Similar to sugar, salt comes in many forms and is added to many packaged foods. So it is not always easy to keep track of how much salt you are consuming. Good sources of salt include plain sea salt, natural tamari soy sauce, miso, and pickled foods such as umeboshi plums, sauerkraut, and cucumber pickles. Sea salt is also found in many natural prepared foods, like crackers and chips, breads, and some roasted nuts. So even if you are on a natural diet, it is quite easy to take in too much. Although salt is an important ingredient in our diet and should *not* be entirely eliminated, neither should it be indulged in. In the macrobiotic diet, pure sea salt is not usually sprinkled on prepared foods. Rather, macrobiotic condiments containing salt are carefully balanced with other ingredients. Too much salt can lead to anemia, excessive thirst, or cravings for sweets or chilled foods. Over a long period of time, too much salt may also contribute to a rigid or stubborn personality. So take care not to overload soup with miso, and avoid pouring tamari soy sauce over all of your foods. Tune into the taste of the *food*, rather than the taste of the seasoning. In general, strive for the middle of the road in your cooking—neither too bland nor too salty—in order to avoid problems caused by either too much or too little salt.

Liquids

Many of us have heard the recommendation that we drink six to eight glasses of water every day. This can cause several problems associated with overworked kidneys, such as a feeling of fatigue and frequent urination. Also, too much liquid dilutes digestive fluids and weakens normal digestive functions. There is no one answer to the question of how much we should drink, for there is no set amount of liquid that is right to drink every day.

Every individual is slightly different. Every day is also slightly different. On hot and dry days, you may require more liquid. On cold and rainy days, you may require less. Some activities may be very physically demanding, using up your stores of liquid rather quickly. Other activities may require less energy, thus calling for less liquid.

There is no sense in gulping down quarts of water or large amounts of juice and tea, just because you think you should. Let your common sense decide how much is right to drink. Remember, though, that if you consume too much salt you'll want to drink more than usual. So go easy on the salt. Unless the weather is very hot, or you are very active, a cup of soup with lunch and dinner and a cup or two of hot tea after meals will provide sufficient liquid for your body. Remember also that vegetables, which constitute a large part of the macrobiotic diet, are naturally juicy, and that grains and beans are generally prepared with more water than foods like meat, cheese, and eggs. Since you are already obtaining a considerable amount of liquid directly from your food, a smaller quantity of beverages is needed.

Baked Foods

Cookies, crusty breads and rolls, chips, crackers, and pastry crusts—they're all delightful to munch on but difficult to digest. Don't deny yourself an occasional cookie or cracker, but understand that too many hard, baked foods can cause problems in your digestive tract. This is true regardless of whether such foods are made from unrefined, whole grain flour or refined, white flour. Baked flour products can also contribute to constipation and to pancreatic and liver problems; therefore, it's best not to eat these foods every day. Whole grains, cracked grains, noodles, and pasta are much easier to digest. However, if you do eat foods that are hard or dry, try combining them with foods that are soft or moist, such as spreads, vegetables, soup, or tea.

Natural Sweets

Although not everyone is born with a "sweet tooth," everyone appreciates sweetness to some degree. Among the foods recommended in the macrobiotic diet is a complete range of sweet-tasting foods. Several grains, especially brown rice, have a natural sweetness when chewed well. Cooked vegetables, such as squash and onions, carrots, turnips, and parsnips, are even more sweet. But if you are used to a lot of sugar it may take time to fully appreciate the sweet flavor of grains and vegetables. Still more sweet are several whole foods that make excellent choices for wholesome desserts. These are *amasake* pudding and *mochi* (both made from whole sweet rice), cooked chestnuts, and fresh, dried, or cooked fruits. You can create many pleasing desserts using these foods. In addition, for added sweetness, try using syrups and powders made from malted grains. With such a full variety of sweet foods, you can satisfy any sweet tooth and create desserts that meet any standard of taste.

Fiber

Today, there is lots of publicity about dietary fiber. Fiber, of course, is essential to the proper functioning of the whole digestive process. But wheat bran and bran products are only necessary in a diet that lacks fiber in the first place—that is, in a diet that is high in refined foods and foods which are completely lacking in fiber, such as meat, eggs, dairy products, and oil. Whole grains and vegetables are both excellent sources of fiber in a macrobiotic diet. By eating a whole foods, natural diet, you will not have to worry about how much processed bran you should eat; rather, you will automatically obtain all the fiber you need from your daily meals.

Overeating

If you find yourself eating more than usual, there

are several possible reasons which you may want to consider.

1. *Too much salt.* An excessive intake of salt can lead to excessive eating. Check your diet to see if you are eating a lot of salty pickles, corn chips, pretzels, crackers, or popcorn, or too much sea salt, miso, or soy sauce. Try reducing your use of these items, but don't eliminate them entirely. If you use no salt at all, you may begin to feel tired, listless, or lacking in appetite. Instead, pay careful attention to the amount of salt you use in preparing foods. This can quickly reduce excessive hunger. However, if your diet has been very salty for many years, it may take several weeks or even months for your appetite to become more moderate.

2. *An unbalanced diet.* An unbalanced diet can also lead to overeating. Excessive hunger may be a sign that something is lacking in your diet. If you find yourself eating constantly, your body may be trying to supply, through sheer *volume*, whatever nutrient is lacking in your diet. For instance, if you overlook protein-rich foods in your diet and eat only grains and vegetables, you may find yourself unconsciously overeating in order to get an adequate supply of protein from the smaller amounts of protein available in grains and vegetables. This can also be true of sweets. If you suddenly deny yourself all sweet foods— even good-quality ones—you may find yourself craving more of everything else. Again, the body may be trying to obtain potassium or some other essential nutrient that it is lacking through quan-

tity. Cravings are your body's way of telling you what it needs. When your diet is adequate, cravings are rare and mild. When your diet becomes careless, however, cravings become stronger and more frequent.

3. *Hypoglycemia.* It has been estimated that over 50% of Americans experience symptoms of hypoglycemia. This condition, which results from a disorder in the pancreas, can lead to overeating and, sometimes, to compulsive eating. If you suspect you have this problem, avoid eating salty foods, as well as baked flour products such as cookies, breads, and crackers (which accelerate pancreatic problems) and emphasize softer, less salty foods in your diet. Lightly-cooked green vegetables are important, as are sea greens, particularly *arame.* An important book for anyone with hypoglycemia is *Diabetes and Hypoglycemia* by Michio Kushi (Japan Publications, 1985).

4. *Sudden changes.* A sudden change in your eating patterns can also cause cravings and overeating. If you suddenly withhold *all* the foods to which you have long been accustomed, such as daily servings of meat, sweets, or dairy foods, your body will quite naturally continue to desire what it is suddenly lacking. Therefore, it helps to withdraw these foods *slowly* in order to give your body time to get used to new foods. Avoid putting your body through sudden and violent changes that will disrupt digestive functions. Changing to a more wholesome way of eating is a little like driving a car. One has to gently let out the clutch while slowly pressing in on the

accelerator. These two actions have to be well coordinated in order for the car to run smoothly. So it is with diet. One must gently relinquish the use of unwholesome foods while slowly increasing the use of more healthful ones.

So check your daily diet to be sure it is adequate and well-balanced, and to see that you are eating a sufficient variety of basic foods every day. You'll find that any problems which occur can usually be traced to a lack of proper proportion among various types of food—for instance, too much bread or too few vegetables—or else to poor cooking skills. Letting out the clutch too fast—in other words, rejecting all of your former foods too suddenly—will only result in a "stalled" car. You may make a few mistakes at first, but once you learn to listen to your body, and to nourish it properly, you'll be cruising along with ease.

Pregnancy

If you are pregnant or are planning on having a baby, you probably already know that pregnancy is an important time for proper nourishment. The food a woman consumes during this period is particularly important to the development of her child. A pregnant woman needs to give extra care to her diet to ensure that she has a healthy child. The quality of nutrition a woman receives during the period *before* conception is also important in determining the quality of her blood, which will directly nourish the new life of her child.

Sugar, honey, and, of course, any kind of hallucinogenic drug should be completely avoided. It is also wise to limit the use of common symptomatic medications for colds, headaches, and so on. Furthermore, be careful in your intake of salt and fruits, and minimize the use of dairy products. Candy bars, donuts, soda, and other junk foods are never advisable, especially during pregnancy. While it is unwise to overly restrict your diet during pregnancy, such a time deserves extra attention to diet, much more so than usual. This special time in your life is crucial to your child's future health and happiness.

Since a mother's diet—before, during, and after pregnancy—is a matter of extreme importance, it is best for couples to prepare themselves for parenting as far in advance as possible. If prospective parents have already adopted a more wholesome way of eating *before* they conceive a child, this can greatly add to the future health and well-being of their child. This is even more true for those who plan on practicing informed natural childbirth and breastfeeding.

An invaluable guide for pregnant mothers and all parents is *Macrobiotic Pregnancy and Care of the Newborn* by Michio and Aveline Kushi (Japan Publications, 1984). It is highly recommended for all parents and future parents as a source of information on infant and child care.

WHERE TO LEARN MORE

Those who have access to a good center for macrobiotic education will find that time spent taking macrobiotic cooking classes is well worth it. Qualified teachers and counsellors at the macrobiotic center will answer many of your questions about various foods and cooking techniques. You will be able to see for yourself how whole foods are used, and you can learn, by tasting, about the correct seasonings and proper flavors for various kinds of new foods. A macrobiotic center is also the best place to learn more about the macrobiotic approach to natural health care. Most centers hold regular seminars on cooking and nutrition, in addition to weekly or bi-weekly dinners, where you can enjoy good macrobiotic meals and meet new friends. There are also "pot luck" dinners in many communities.

If you do not have a macrobiotic center in your area, you might want to visit one in another city, or attend one of the many week-long macrobiotic summer seminars in the United States or Canada. Even one week-end at a good macrobiotic center can help you discover new dietary choices and deepen your awareness of what you eat. It can also put you in touch with others in your area who share similar interests. Most centers have mailing lists, which may help you to locate smaller macrobiotic groups or individual friends—along with natural foods stores and restaurants—in your area.

There are also many good books available now on the subject of macrobiotics—not only excellent cookbooks, but also books on natural macrobiotic health care. You can order these by mail if your local bookstore or natural foods store does not already carry them. A list of resources for macrobiotic learning and further information may also be found in Appendix C.

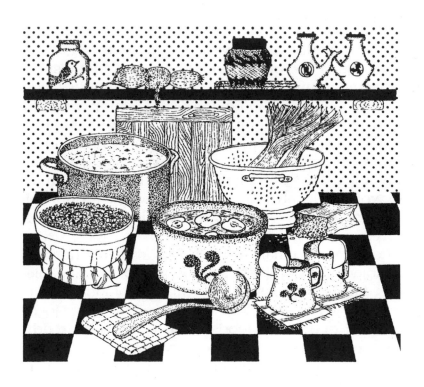

5

The Most Important Point

The key to success with a macrobiotic diet lies in learning how to cook well, for natural foods can be either delicious or unappetizing, depending on how they are prepared. Cookbooks, of course, can be very helpful, but nothing can compare with direct instruction from a competent cooking instructor. Once you learn good cooking skills, eating natural foods will become a pleasure. The feeling that results from consuming wholesome, delicious meals on a daily basis has to be experienced in order to be truly appreciated.

Poor cooking skills, in fact, are the most common handicap that people experience when beginning a macrobiotic diet. This is because most of us have never cooked foods such as whole grains (barley, brown rice, millet, etc.) As a result, we know nothing about how much water or salt to add, nor the various interesting ways there are to season such foods.

Even familiar foods like vegetables are often poorly cooked —this is one reason why children often do not enjoy them. Except for raw salads, many of us haven't ventured too far beyond frozen peas and carrots, or canned corn and string beans. How far removed these dull preparations are from the succulent flavors of a piping hot stir-fry, or the crisp tartness of homemade pickles. Even plain, lightly-steamed, fresh vegetables are much more appealing in taste and texture than frozen and canned vegetables.

People are often tempted to introduce unsuspecting kin to natural foods when their cooking skills are still at a beginner's level. This experience can alienate your family from natural foods forever. Culinary disasters like this can be avoided if you learn some simple ways to make meals appetizing and attractive. As with any other type of cuisine, macrobiotic foods are dependent upon the cook's ability to capture their taste and enhance their appeal during the transformation that is undergone in the kitchen.

In fairness to the cook, however, it is also true that the more gentle tastes of natural foods are often too subtle, initially, for jaded palates and tastebuds numbed by continual exposure to excessive salt, sugar, and spices. But, in time, this sensitivity will return, as cooking skills improve and meals become the satisfying and delicious experiences they should be.

If you should burn the beans or ruin the rice when first starting out, don't become discouraged. These are problems that everyone encounters at first, so stay relaxed when you are in the kitchen, and *persevere*. Don't give up during the first few weeks, while you're still learning new tastes and new cooking techniques. Instead, give yourself *time.*

PLANNING MEALS

In deciding *what to cook* for a particular meal, the important thing to remember is *variety.* A well-balanced meal generally includes at least one whole grain food, a protein food, and several kinds of freshly-cooked vegetables (including greens and sea greens). Various garnishes and condiments also add interest and balance to a meal, and salad or pickles contribute a note of freshness. This kind of variety will help you to achieve a good balance of tastes, textures, and nutrients.

One good way to plan a meal is to select the grain dish first—such as brown rice, millet croquettes, or wheat pilaf—then build the rest of the meal around this central dish. Next, choose a protein food to suit the grain you have selected. Add at least two different vegetable dishes of contrasting colors and types, such as roots, heads, or greens (and sea greens) to round out the meal. Then select a soup that harmonizes with your menu thus far, and choose the garnishes that will add a bright touch to the meal or vary its texture, such as finely-chopped scallions or parsley, toasted sesame or sunflower seeds, etc.

By following this general plan, you can create a well-rounded meal that is rich in variety. Stocking your shelves with jars of grains, beans, noodles, seeds, nuts, dried vegetables, fruits, and sea greens will show you at a glance the various choices open to you for a meal. But be aware that variety is also seen in the frequency with which you prepare each dish. A certain food might be healthful, interesting, and delicious when served on occasion, but it can quickly lose its appeal if you serve it three nights a week. Similarly, a particular menu—well-balanced and pleasing though it may be—may lose its appeal if you serve it over and over again. (For staple foods such as brown rice, which you may want to repeat often, you can always add a touch of something different to keep it "interesting," such as barley, millet, fresh corn or peas, etc.) Good cooking does not consist of learning a set number of recipes. Rather, it is the art of adapting menus to daily and seasonal cycles. But good health and satisfaction *cannot* be maintained without variety. A good cook; therefore, is inventive and imaginative—within reason, of course—and will vary the menu from day to day, week to week, and season to season.

In deciding *how to cook* what you have selected, the key here is *contrast*. Contrast can be expressed in many different ways, primarily through the use of different *cooking techniques, seasonings,* and *time.*

Cooking Techniques

In preparing vegetables, don't limit yourself to merely boiling and steaming, or only frying and baking. You and your family will soon tire of eating foods prepared in only one or two different ways, and your meals as a whole will become dull and unappetizing. To create interesting meals, use two or three different styles of cooking *in one meal*—baking, boiling, stir-frying, sautéing, stewing, steaming, pressure-cooking, etc. This will provide sufficient contrast to impart a feeling of satisfaction. Avoid making too many steamed, fried, or boiled dishes, and so on.

Salt, Water, Oil, & Other Seasonings

The amount of salt, water, oil, and other seasonings you use can also help to create interesting contrasts within a meal. For example, some foods taste best when they are slightly salty, while others taste better salt-free. Some dishes require more water, such as soups, stews, and sauces, while others need little or no water, such as stir-fried vegetables, baked winter squash, and tempura. By keeping these things in mind when you cook, you will be able to create interesting contrasts in your meals.

Time

Another kind of contrast can be achieved by varying dishes that are cooked for a *long* time with those that are cooked a *short* time. Certain foods—such as beans, root vegetables, and some sea greens—are best when simmered slowly for an hour or more to bring out a full, rich, flavor and hearty quality. Other foods, usually the lighter kinds of vegetables, are best when lightly-cooked—steamed, blanched, or par-boiled—or when they are served raw in the form of pickles or salad.

An example of a good meal is one which includes a "strong" dish, such as a well-cooked root vegetable stew or a slowly-simmered bean dish; a fresher, lighter food, such as steamed vegetables, salad, or quick pickles; something prepared without oil, such as noodles or pressure-cooked grains; and, occasionally, something else prepared with a touch of oil, such as a sautéed vegetable.

Too many protein dishes (for example, beans *and* fish), too many water-based dishes (soup *and* stew), or too many well-cooked dishes will make a meal both less balanced and less appealing. The reverse is also true. If a meal doesn't have any protein dish, it may leave you feeling unsatisfied, even though you have eaten a sufficient amount of food. If a meal is too dry, without any softer texture or consistency, it may be less appetizing than it could be. If a meal, taken as a whole, is too lightly-cooked—with nothing to "stick to your ribs"—more care is necessary in selecting and preparing your menus. It helps to check your menu *before* you begin to cook, to be sure that it is hearty enough to be satisfying, yet not too heavy. Obviously, you needn't run through this litany at every meal, but because the period when first trying to cook a new cuisine can be awkward, it helps to learn different ways of creating balance, contrast, and variety.

As you gain experience, balanced cooking will come "naturally" and satisfying meals will be the result. Common sense and intuition are preferable to a conceptual approach in the kitchen, but in the beginning it is important to learn the basics and to gain a good understanding of macrobiotic dietary principles. These valuable guidelines are available in macrobiotic books and courses, which every cook, experienced or beginner, should review periodically.

Another goal to strive for is that of satisfying those for whom you cook, *whose needs may be different from yours.* Ask family members what natural foods they enjoy most, and prepare their favorites often. One person may enjoy a little more salt, while another may like a little less. One may enjoy sweet-tasting dishes, while another may want more salad or fish. This doesn't mean making separate meals every day—it just means making adjustments in the weekly menu by adding an extra dish here and there.

It also helps to keep a variety of fresh salad vegetables on hand. Many new cooks tend to ignore the
importance of lighter foods, and salad alleviates the
"overcooked vegetables syndrome" until you develop
some expertise in preparing lighter, fresher vegetable
dishes. Also, by expanding your cooking skills to include cooking techniques from other countries, you
will be able to create pleasing and interesting menus
every day of the week. If your family prefers only
American-style meals, then oblige them, creatively,
with hearty wheat-meat stews, their favorite soups,
baked beans, fried fish, coleslaw, onion rings, fruit
salads, puddings, pies, vegetarian chili, tempeh
"steaks," seitan "cutlets," roasted ears of corn, fish
chowders, soyburgers, and so forth. It can be both
challenging and fun to prepare familiar dishes in
healthier ways.

Do try to avoid slipping into a hasty cuisine (even
if it's an all-natural one) composed of meals that are
too simple and inadequate instead of balanced and
well-rounded. This is not the way to longevity and
health. Make it a priority to devote sufficient time
and energy to preparing your daily meals. While it
may require some concessions to our hectic, modern
lifestyles, it is still possible, even with a limited amount
of time, to prepare wholesome meals. This is another
reason for studying macrobiotic cooking with a competent instructor. You will learn the various ways
others have discovered to overcome the obstacle of
"too little time."

Granted, the days of sitting on the veranda and
snapping green beans are a thing of the past, and
most of us have jobs that don't allow for much time
in the kitchen. But by organizing your kitchen and
streamlining meal preparation, you can prepare delicious, nutritious meals within a reasonable amount

of time. Recruit other family members to wash and slice vegetables. Cut down on kitchen time in other ways by planning menus ahead of time and shopping in advance, so you will have everything you need on hand.

Don't allow yourself to slide into poor eating habits, slipshod meals, or reliance on too many convenience foods—even those purchased from a health food store. Chips, sandwiches, cookies, instant soups, instant noodles, etc. are only a few steps away from junk food. Short-cuts like these don't work. Diet deserves a certain amount of time and attention. The sooner you recognize this fact, the sooner you can establish a routine that works for you. Remember— everything has its price, and good health requires more than just setting the dial on the microwave.

In time, you will find that the rewards are well worth the effort. In fact, the time and energy you invest in practicing good habits of cooking and eating will equal the degree of health and well-being that you enjoy.

It is obvious, therefore, that learning how to cook well is a matter of the highest importance. It is the key to success with macrobiotics. Even when you learn the basics, never stop learning; keep on adding to your repertoire through classes and books, and by exchanging ideas with friends.

All in all, there are *three main points* to remember when beginning a macrobiotic diet.

1. *Go slowly but perseveringly.* Emulate the patient and persevering turtle, rather than the quick and seemingly-successful hare. Go steadily, one step at a time.

2. *Learn to cook well. Take* the time to cook. *Make the time to cook.* In the long run, your life and health depend on it.

3. *Eventually move beyond a transitional diet.* Remember that a transitional diet is only a stepping-stone from an unhealthy diet to a healthful one. While it is much healthier than a meat-dairy-and-sugar diet, it is not a way of eating that can bring truly good health. The length of time that you will need a transitional diet will vary; for some it will be months, for others it may be years. But at some point move on to the *standard macrobiotic diet* if you wish to experience your optimum level of health and well-being.

At first, making the change to a macrobiotic diet may seem like a rather big adjustment in your life. It certainly requires a little more time and forethought than your former diet entailed. But thousands of people are making this adjustment for the sake of their health, and those who have are glad they did. The choice is one you will never regret if you practice it correctly, because although good food brings good results slowly, it brings them surely. When all is said and done, you'll undoubtedly find, as many others have, that a macrobiotic diet isn't always the most convenient diet in the world—it's simply the *best*!

Appendices

A. Common Questions

Without citrus fruits, what is the source of Vitamin C in a macrobiotic diet?

There are many good sources of Vitamin C besides oranges, such as broccoli, brussel sprouts, cabbage, cantaloupe, cauliflower, collard greens, kale, mustard greens, parsley, strawberries, turnip greens, watercress, and watermelon.

What can I use in place of sugar?

There are many more wholesome sweeteners available—barley-malt syrup, rice syrup, rice syrup powder, fresh fruit, dried fruit, fruit purées, and fruit butters such as apple or apricot. While making the transition to a macrobiotic diet, you may also want to use maple syrup temporarily.

What is a good source of iron in a macrobiotic diet?

There are many rich sources of iron among the foods recommended in a macrobiotic diet, such as dried beans (especially aduki beans and soy beans), buckwheat noodles, and miso soup. Other particularly good sources of iron are found among green vegetables, sea greens, and shellfish.

From where is iodine obtained if not from iodized salt?

Sea salt is approximately 90-94% sodium chloride. The remainder consists of various trace minerals, including iodine. Iodine is also plentiful in both sea greens and seafood.

What is the source of calcium in a macrobiotic diet?

Dark green, leafy vegetables (collards, kale, mustard greens, turnip greens, carrot tops, etc.) are excellent sources of calcium. Calcium is also provided by sea greens, fish and seafood, seeds and nuts, and many beans (especially soy beans).

Is there any danger of becoming anemic in a macrobiotic diet?

It is possible to become anemic on *any* kind of diet, if you do not eat proper meals. For example, filling up on too many snack foods such as rice cakes, crackers, chips, or cookies and skipping such nourishing and sustaining foods as miso soup, green vegetables, protein foods, and sea greens can definitely lead to a deficiency condition. In this way, you deprive your body of essential nutrients.

Eating insufficient variety, over-salting foods, or over-cooking foods can all contribute to an anemic condition. Therefore, it is important to distinguish between a misinformed, or incorrect practice of a macrobiotic diet, and a correct or proper practice of a macrobiotic diet.

Similarly, parents who give their children too many baked flour products (such as cookies, crackers, and breads), or who are not careful in regulating the amount of salt and variety of foods (especially green vegetables) in their children's diets, may be contributing to the development of rickets in their children. Such slovenly habits can lead to a distortion of the macrobiotic diet and often give the true macrobiotic diet a bad reputation.

If I don't like sea greens, where can I get minerals from?

Dark, leafy greens (collards, kale, mustard greens, turnip greens, carrot tops, etc.) are all rich in minerals. However, sea greens are an important element of a macrobiotic diet. Do not get discouraged if you do not find them appealing at first, for they are not a familiar food in our culture. *Your tastes will change in time*, and as you learn how to prepare them properly you will be surprised to find that they can be a very delicious addition to your diet.

Aren't carbohydrates fattening?

Obesity is not common among people who consume grains as a principle food. However, *refined* starches, such as white bread, white rice, white noodles, and so on, *can* mean extra pounds. These processed foods tend to increase our appetites for other foods, rather than satisfy us as whole foods do.

From where is Vitamin B-12 obtained?

Vitamin B-12 can be obtained from fish and sea-food, as well as from some sea vegetables and certain fermented soy bean products, such as miso and tamari. Tempeh is also a good source of B-12 when it is made correctly.

B. Glossary

Amasake (ah-ma-za-kee). A sweet made from whole grains that can be served as a pudding or a drink, depending on the consistency. It is usually made from the fermentation of sweet rice, and may be flavored with fresh or cooked fruits. It can be served warm or cool, according to the season. Though it is sold as both a liquid and a concentrate, you can also make it easily yourself if it is not yet available in your area. Commercial amasakes vary considerably in quality. Purchase only those made from *whole* sweet brown rice rather than those made from white rice or those which have other questionable ingredients in them.

Kuzu (koo-zoo). Comes in small white chunks that quickly dissolve in cold water. It is used as a thickener—like cornstarch or arrowroot—for sauces, gravies, and puddings.

Miso (mee-so). A highly nutritious concentrate made from soy beans and grains. The flavor and quality of miso vary according to the ingredients and the length of the fermentation process. Pure soy bean miso has a rather strong taste, while miso made with barley or rice has a milder flavor. Miso is used primarily for seasoning soups, and miso soup is an important part of a macrobiotic diet because of the rich nutrients it provides. Properly-aged barley miso (at least eighteen months) is a good choice for general use. Miso is rich in protein, Vitamin B-12, and various enzymes which aid in digestion. Natural, unpasteurized miso is best.

Mochi (moh-chee). Traditionally made by pounding whole-cooked sweet rice until it becomes glutinous. It is then allowed to dry in the cold air and harden. This is then prepared by pan-toasting or baking briefly in the oven, at which time it puffs up into soft, chewy treats. Depending on how it is prepared, mochi can be served as a main course, a snack, or as a dessert.

Sea Greens. Dried sea vegetables. At harvest, they are usually rinsed and laid out in the sun to dry. There is a wide range of sea greens in the coastal waters around the world. Sea greens are a rich source of minerals as well as vitamins. Some sea greens are best only in soups or as side dishes, while others can be easily incorporated into almost any kind of dish.

Agar Agar (ah-gar ah-gar). Also called "angels hair," it is tasteless and neutral in color. It is used to make

a cool and refreshing gelatin-like dessert called kan-
ten. It can be flavored with fruit juice and/or fruits,
or used in vegetable aspics flavored by a seasoned
vegetable broth and shredded vegetables.

Arame. A dark, shredded sea vegetable. Mild and
sweet in flavor, it is usually prepared as a side dish
with onions or onions and carrots.

Dulse. A sea vegetable found on American shores
that was traditionally used by native Americans. It
can be lightly roasted, crushed, and used as a condiment, or rinsed and used raw in salads. Dulse is also
a good source of Vitamin C.

Hiziki (hee-zee-kee). A very dark, fibrous sea green,
rather strong in taste. It is best when gently simmered
for at least an hour, using carrots and onions to
sweeten it, and it is often seasoned with tamari soy
sauce and toasted sesame or sunflower seeds. Rich
in iron and other minerals, it makes a nourishing
side dish.

Irish Moss. Native to the shores of Ireland, Irish
moss is akin to agar agar and similar in use.

Kombu (kom-boo). Dark green strips of kombu are
used to make soup stock, to soften beans, to sweeten
root vegetables such as carrots, or as a condiment.
It is similar to native American kelp.

Nori. Comes packaged in delicate paper-thin sheets.
It is lightly toasted on a gas flame until it turns a
lighter shade of green. Then it can be wrapped
around rice and vegetables (nori rolls) or rice and
fish (sushi) as a kind of sandwich. It can also be

crumbled over soups and noodles as a condiment. Akin to native American laver, nori is a good source of iron—especially ao-nori, or nori flakes.

Wakame (wa-ka-may). A green sea vegetable that cooks quickly and is used in soups, salads, and side dishes, or toasted and crushed to make a condiment. Wakame is also a rich source of calcium.

Tamari (ta-ma-ree). A natural soy sauce that does not contain the chemical additives or sugar often found in other kinds of soy sauce. It can be used to flavor soups, vegetables, noodles, fried rice, and many other dishes, where it imparts a rich and slightly salty flavor.

Tempeh (tem-pay). A traditional Indonesian food, tempeh is made by a process involving the fermentation of whole soy beans, which results in a cheese-like texture. Tempeh is used like meat in stews, soups, sandwiches, and kebabs, and makes a hearty, filling food. Tempeh that is not fresh can be bitter or soggy when cooked, so be sure that the tempeh you buy is as fresh as possible.

Tofu. Having also originated in the Orient, tofu has a lighter texture than tempeh and a neutral flavor. This makes it adaptable to many different kinds of recipes and seasonings. It can be used in soups, stews, salads, casseroles, and many other dishes—either boiled, steamed, or deep-fried. Tofu spoils or sours very quickly, so it should be purchased only when fresh and used within a day or two of purchasing.

Umeboshi. Small, pickled plums with a salty-sour taste. They are used as a condiment with rice or wherever a sour taste is desired, such as in salad dressings.

Wheat meat (also called **seitan**). Originally from China, wheat meat is a meat-like vegetable protein made from whole wheat flour, which is then cooked and seasoned with tamari soy sauce. Wheat meat is often thinly sliced for use in sandwiches or cubed for use in stews and kebabs.

C. Recommended Reading

GENERAL READING

- *The Macrobiotic Way* by Michio Kushi, Avery Publishing Group, 1985
- *The Natural Shopper's Guide* by Dan Seamens and David Wollner, East West Journal, 1982
- *An Introduction To Macrobiotics* by Carolyn Heidenry, Aladdin Press, 1984

COOKBOOKS

- *The Changing Seasons Macrobiotic Cookbook* by Aveline Kushi and Wendy Esko, Avery Publishing Group, 1985
- *The Whole World Cookbook, International Macrobiotic Cuisine,* Avery Publishing Group, 1984
- *The Book of Whole Meals* by Annemarie Colbin, Ballantine Books, 1979

For those who wish to study further, the Kushi Institute, an educational institution founded in Boston in 1979 with affiliates in London, Amsterdam, and Antwerp, offers full- and part-time instruction for individuals who wish to become macrobiotic teachers and counselors. The Kushi Institute publishes a "Macrobiotic Teachers and Counselors Directory," listing graduates who are qualified to offer guidance in the macrobiotic approach to health.

> **Kushi Institute**
> **P.O. Box 7**
> **Becket, MA 01223**
> **(413) 623-5741**

Ongoing developments in macrobiotics are reported in various publications, including the *East West Journal*, a monthly magazine begun in 1971 and now with an international readership of 200,000. The *EWJ* features regular articles on the macrobiotic approach to health and nutrition, as well as ecology, science, psychology, the arts, and pregnancy, natural birth, and child care.

> ***East West Journal***
> **17 Station Street**
> **Brookline, MA 02147**
> **(617) 232-1000**

D. Major Mail-Order Companies for Natural Foods

Granum
2901 NE Blakely Street
Seattle, WA 98105
(206) 525-0051

Macrobiotic Wholesale Company
503 Haywood Road
Asheville, NC 28806
800-438-4730

Mountain Ark Trading Co.
120 SE Avenue
Fayetteville, AR 72701
800-643-8909

Oak Feed Store
3030 Grand Avenue
Coconut Grove, Miami, FL 33133
(305) 448-7595

Ohsawa America
P.O. Box 3068
Chico, CA 95927
(916) 342-6050

SHOPPING

VEGETABLES

☐ Acorn Squash
☐ Bok Choy
☐ Broccoli
☐ Brussel Sprouts
☐ Burdock
☐ Buttercup Squash
☐ Butternut Squash
☐ Cabbage
☐ Carrot Tops
☐ Carrots
☐ Cauliflower
☐ Celery
☐ Chinese Cabbage
☐ Collard Greens
☐ Crookneck Squash
☐ Cucumber
☐ Daikon
☐ Endive
☐ Hubbard Squash
☐ Kale
☐ Leeks
☐ Lettuce
☐ Lotus Root
☐ Mushrooms
☐ Mustard Greens
☐ Onions
☐ Parsley
☐ Parsnips
☐ Peas
☐ Pumpkin
☐ Radishes
☐ Red Cabbage
☐ Rutabaga
☐ Scallions
☐ Sprouts
☐ String Beans
☐ Swiss Chard
☐ Turnip Greens
☐ Turnips
☐ Watercress

WHOLE GRAINS

☐ Barley
☐ Brown Rice
☐ Buckwheat
☐ Corn (whole)
☐ Millet
☐ Oats
☐ Rye
☐ Sweet Rice
☐ Wheat

BEANS & BEAN PRODUCTS

☐ Aduki Beans
☐ Black Soy Beans
☐ Black Turtle Beans
☐ Chick Peas (Garbanzo)
☐ Great Northern Beans
☐ Kidney Beans
☐ Lentils
☐ Navy Beans
☐ Pinto Beans
☐ Red Lentils
☐ Tofu
☐ Tempeh
☐ Soy Beans
☐ Split Peas
☐ Wheat Meat

SWEETENERS

☐ Apple Butter
☐ Barley Malt
☐ Currants
☐ Dried Apples
☐ Dried Apricots
☐ Dried Peaches
☐ Dried Pears
☐ Maple Syrup
☐ Raisins
☐ Rice Syrup

LIST

GRAIN PRODUCTS

- ☐ Bread (whole grain flour)
- ☐ Bulghur
- ☐ Cornmeal
- ☐ Couscous
- ☐ Cracked Wheat
- ☐ Flour (whole grain)
- ☐ Mochi
- ☐ Noodles & Pasta (whole grain)
- ☐ Oatmeal
- ☐ Rolled Wheat, Rye or Barley Flakes
- ☐ Steel-cut Oats

SEA GREENS

- ☐ Agar Agar
- ☐ Arame
- ☐ Dulse
- ☐ Hiziki
- ☐ Irish Moss
- ☐ Kelp
- ☐ Kombu
- ☐ Laver
- ☐ Nori
- ☐ Wakame

FRUITS

- ☐ Apples
- ☐ Apricots
- ☐ Blueberries
- ☐ Cantaloupe
- ☐ Cherries
- ☐ Chestnuts
- ☐ Grapes
- ☐ Peaches
- ☐ Pears
- ☐ Plums
- ☐ Raspberries
- ☐ Strawberries
- ☐ Watermelon

SPECIALTY ITEMS

- ☐ Kuzu
- ☐ Shitake Mushrooms

SEASONINGS

- ☐ Corn Oil
- ☐ Ginger Root
- ☐ Mirin
- ☐ Miso
- ☐ Sea Salt
- ☐ Sesame Oil
- ☐ Tamari Soy Sauce
- ☐ Umeboshi Plums
- ☐ Umeboshi Vinegar
- ☐ Vinegar (Brown Rice)

SNACKS

- ☐ Cookies
- ☐ Corn Chips
- ☐ Crackers
- ☐ Granola
- ☐ Muesli
- ☐ Muffins
- ☐ Peanut Butter
- ☐ Popcorn
- ☐ Rice Cakes
- ☐ Sesame Butter
- ☐ Tahini

BEVERAGES

- ☐ Amasake
- ☐ Barley Tea
- ☐ Fruit Juice
- ☐ Grain Coffee
- ☐ Herb Tea
- ☐ Kukicha Tea
- ☐ Spring Water

SEEDS & NUTS

- ☐ Almonds
- ☐ Peanuts
- ☐ Pecans
- ☐ Pumpkin Seeds
- ☐ Sesame Seeds
- ☐ Sunflower Seeds
- ☐ Walnuts

Index